Praying Through Lyme Disease

BOOK OF PRAYERS
2ND EDITION
LARGE PRINT EDITION

REBECCA VANDEMARK

dedication

to my mom, my best friend, who taught
me the joy of praying through trials, and
to my dad, my hero, who has spent
countless hours on his knees on my
behalf.

acknowledgments

All scripture in this book has been noted or referenced in this book. There have been numerous versions used to help encourage the reader to look at a variety of different scriptural references in their journey. May you find rest, encouragement, and hope in the living and active word of God and prayer.

"Come and hear, all you who fear God, let me tell you what He has done for me. I cried out to Him with my mouth, His praise was on my tongue. If I had cherished sin in my heart, the Lord would not have listened, but God has surely heard my prayer. Praise be to God, who has not rejected my prayer or withheld his love from me!"
-Psalm 66:16-20-

content

preface

At a recent Lyme disease conference it was stated that "Lyme disease is the growing epidemic and health crisis of the 21st century"[i] and that "In the fullness of time the mainstream handling of Chronic Lyme Disease will be viewed as one of the most shameful episodes in the history of medicine"[ii]. While not well known, and maybe not well handled in mainstream dialogue, there are hundreds of thousands of Lyme Warriors that struggle each day just to live.

Many of them cannot get out of bed due to extreme and debilitating fatigue and pain. Many are lying in hospital beds with doctors who don't know what to do. Many others are struggling emotionally under the weight of loss. Many others feel completely isolated and forsaken. In the midst of all of this there is a voice and a helper that calls through the dark night and says that He will never abandon or forsaken us. In the midst of sickness and pain it is hard to sometimes know how to pray through the Scriptures of the Bible.

This little book is designed with 31 topics that Lyme disease patients struggle with and verses to meditate on and pray through in times of difficulty and in good days. This book is meant to be a companion and an encouragement to all who are struggling with Lyme disease and the intensity in of their fight.

a note from the author

Dear Fellow Lyme Warrior,

The book that you hold in your hand has been written from my heart. I found out I had Advanced Late Stage Lyme disease the day after my 33rd birthday. For the previous six years prior to that day I had experienced a myriad of intricate and confusing health symptoms that never made sense to any doctor. I had spent hundreds of hours traveling across the United States talking and consulting with some of the best in the country. No answers came and I was eventually told that either (a) this was "in my head", (b) I had a very "complex case" of Chronic Fatigue Syndrome (for which I had been diagnosed for) or (c) "stress was contributing to these issues". Finally, after seeing 273 doctors in one year, seven years of searching, hundreds of invasive and painful tests, and thousands of prayers, I was correctly and accurately diagnosed with Advanced Late Stage Lyme disease. While my family and I rejoiced that there was finally an answer, I also experienced a range of emotions as I was furious with the medical community and overwhelmed with where to go from that point on.

During this time and since then, there are so many times where it is hard to know what to pray except for "please Lord, heal me" and yet (as with everything with Lyme Disease) I have found that there are so many emotions and issues that accompany Lyme Disease beyond that simple cry of my heart. Out of this journey has come the book that you are reading. My prayer with this book is that it will encourage you, lead you to Scripture, and remind you that you are not alone in this fight. The journey is long and yet the Lord is near. I pray that this book is a jump start for your prayer life through this disease.

There are 31 topics covered in this book to match the days of the months of the year. Feel free to go in order or to skip around to what is most on your heart. The word of God is living and active and I pray that you find Scriptures that you can pray through that speak to your specific hearts needs. With each topic there is also a section of "prayer notes" where you can record your own prayers and Scriptures and where you can visibly see how the Lord is answering the prayers of your heart day after day, month after month, and year after year.

May the Lord bless you abundantly dear friend and give you strength for the journey before you.

Blessings,
Rebecca

"May the Lord answer you when you are in distress; may the name of the God of Jacob protect you. May He send you help from the sanctuary and grant you support from Zion. May He remember all of your sacrifices and accept your burnt offerings. May He give you the desire of your heart and make all of your plans succeed. May we shout for joy over your victory and lift up our banners in the name of our God. May the Lord grant all of your requests."
-Psalm 20:1-5-

the diagnosis

"Even though I walk through the
darkest valley, I will not be afraid, for
you are close beside me."
-Psalm 23:4-

Lord, the news of this diagnosis of
Lyme disease has overwhelmed my
heart. I know that *"yea, though I walk
through the valley of the shadow of death, I will
fear no evil; for You are with me; Your rod and
Your staff, they comfort me."* (Psalm 23:4) I
feel that I am walking in the shadow of
death because this diagnosis
overwhelms me. I am so grateful to
know the answer to the scary symptoms
that I have been experiencing, but
please, Lord, comfort my shaky heart.
Scripture promises that *"the Lord will go
before me and that the God of Israel is my rear
guard"* (Isaiah 52:12). I am not alone in
this fight before me. Lord, while I feel
that everything around me has changed,
I know that your covenant of peace is

with me. Even in the news of this diagnosis I trust you, Lord. I trust your word. *"The mountains may move, and the hills may shake, but my kindness will never depart from you. My promise of peace will never change' says the Lord, who has compassion on you."* (Isaiah 54:10, GOD'S WORD) Amen.

the diagnosis
prayer notes

_____

_____

_____

_____

_____

_____

_____

_____

_____

_____

_____

_____

_____

confusion over treatment options

"Think over what I say, for the Lord
will give you understanding in
everything."
-2 Timothy 2:7-

Lord, one of the hardest parts of this
journey is knowing which treatment
plan is the best for my body. So many
doctors, friends, family members, and
others have so many thoughts on what
to do, but I am confused, Lord.
Scripture states that *"you are not a God of
confusion but of peace"* (I Corinthians
14:33) and I need that peace, Lord. I
trust, Lord that even though *"we are
afflicted in every way, we are not crushed, we
are perplexed but we are not driven to despair"*
(2 Corinthians 4:8) because you, God,
lead us each step that we take. I trust
that the treatment direction that I take
will only help me heal and beat Lyme
disease. I trust that it will not harm me,
but only benefit me because Jesus says,

"nothing shall by any means hurt you" (Luke 10:19). At the end of the day, Lord, I move forward knowing that *"you will give understanding in everything"* (2 Timothy 2:7). Amen.

confusion over treatment options prayer notes

_____

_____

_____

_____

_____

_____

_____

_____

_____

_____

_____

_____

_____

_____

_____

wisdom for doctors

"If any of you needs wisdom to know what you should do, you should ask God, and He will give it to you. God is generous…"
-James1:5, GOD'S WORD-

Lord, I pray for every doctor and physician that I see that you would give them wisdom in how to best help my case. You say in your word that "*if any of you lacks wisdom, let him ask of God, who gives generously and without reproach and it will be given to him*" (James 1:5). I pray, Lord, that you would give wisdom and direct my steps as I move forward (Proverbs 3:5-7). For every medical team member that I see I pray you would give them specific understanding about my case and understanding about how to best help me heal. I pray Lord that *"you would fill them with knowledge"* (Colossians 1:9). I also pray that you would abundantly bless them as they work hard to help me during my time of suffering. *"May they be blessed by the Lord, the Maker of heaven and earth"* (Psalm 115:15). Amen.

wisdom for doctors
prayer notes

_____

_____

_____

_____

_____

_____

_____

_____

_____

_____

_____

_____

feeling discouraged over medical care

"She had suffered a great deal from many doctors and over the years she had spent everything she had to pay them, but she had gotten no better. In fact, she had gotten worse."
-Mark 5:26-

Lord, sometimes when I have to see "other" doctors or those in the medical profession who are not familiar with Lyme disease, I walk out of their office feeling extremely discouraged. I know that I need their expertise to help me with issues that have arisen but it can be discouraging to hear their uninformed criticism of Lyme disease. Their words often cut and are extremely discouraging in light of all that I am dealing with in this journey. Just like the woman in the gospel of Mark, I feel that I have suffered much under many physicians. *"She had suffered much under many physicians,*

17

and had spent all that she had, and was no better but rather grew worse." (Mark 5:26) Lord, I am seeking help from physicians, but I am mostly seeking your help Lord. Help me to remember that these doctors I see are only human, Lord. While they might not understand Lyme disease, you do, Lord. I don't need to be discouraged by their lack of knowledge because you are the all knowing God. Lead me to the medical practitioners who can help me in my healing journey, Lord, and help me to forget those who have spoken discouraging words over me. Help me not to be discouraged by any medical care, but help me to rest in the truth that you are the great physician (John 5:1-9). Amen.

feeling discouraged over medical care prayer notes

_____

_____

_____

_____

_____

_____

_____

_____

_____

_____

_____

_____

_____

_____

feeling like a burden

"They couldn't bring him to Jesus because of the crowd, so they dug a hole through the roof above his head. Then they lowered the man on his mat, right down in front of Jesus."
-Mark 2:4-

Lord, as I fight Lyme I often feel like a burden to those who love me and take care of me each day. During difficult health days it is hard to see the look of pity and sadness on my loved ones faces and hard not to be able to wipe the fatigue of this battle out of their eyes. I know that they love me, Lord, but I often feel like a burden. I feel like a burden as I know that the fight of Lyme disease is a drain on everyone- emotionally, physically, and financially. I see the exhaustion that helping me brings both emotionally and physically, Lord, and I see the quickly dwindling financial resources. I feel like the crowds of necessities for fighting this disease are pushing in around me Lord just like the sick man in the gospel of Mark. And just like the love of the friends of this sick man, my loved ones do everything they can to bring me to where you are. (Mark 2:4) Help me to remember, Lord, that I am not a burden and that you have promised to take care of me and my loved ones. *"Give your burdens to the Lord, and he will take care of you. He will not permit the godly to slip and fall."* (Psalm 55:22) Amen.

feeling like a burden
prayer notes

guilt over how little i am able to do

"Yet if anyone suffers as a Christian, let him not be ashamed, but let him glorify God in that name."
-I Peter 4:16

Lord, in this fast paced and driven world, I often struggle with guilt over needing to rest or stay in bed due to Lyme disease. Sometimes, Lord, the biggest accomplishment that I feel I have had is the ability to sit up in bed for the day. Compared to things that I was able to do in the past and things I feel like I was able to accomplish for your glory this seems like a failure. I struggle as I hear of others who seem to be able to do so much for you because they are healthy Lord. I often take what others are able to do as the measurement for what I should be doing and this makes me feel guilty over how little I am able to do. But, Lord, I know that I am not to compare myself to another. You say in Scripture to *"pay careful attention to your own work, for then you will get satisfaction of a job well done, and you won't need to compare yourself to anyone else"* (Galatians 6:4). Lord, when I stop comparing myself to others and my past, I am able to see clearly the race set before me. *"Therefore, since we are surrounded by such a huge crowd of witnesses to the life of faith, let us strip off every weight that slows us down…and let us run with endurance the race God has set before us."* (Hebrews 12:1) Help me to "run" this race, Lord, for your glory and for you alone. This isn't about *me* Lord, it is all about *you*. I don't need to feel guilt, Lord, because I am not ashamed as I glorify you in this path you have set before me. *"However, if you suffer as a Christian do not be ashamed, but praise God that you bear that name."* (I Peter 4:16) Amen.

guilt over how little i am able to do prayer notes

_____

_____

_____

_____

_____

_____

_____

_____

_____

_____

_____

_____

weakness

"…As thy days are, so shall thy strength
be."
-Deuteronomy 33:25-

Lord, today I am feeling so weak that I
don't think I can even lift my head. This
weakness is so debilitating that it is
impossible to function. You promise,
Lord, that *"as thy days are, so shall thy
strength be"* (Deuteronomy 33:25) and I
am clinging to that promise today. *"It is
you God who arms me with strength and keeps
my way secure."* (Psalm 18:32). It is you,
God, that arms me with strength for this
battle with Lyme disease. *"You have
armed me with strength for the battle…"*
(Psalm 18:39). It is through you, Lord,
alone that I know that I am not defeated
by this weakness because you have given
me today, so you will give me the
strength for it. Guard my mind and
heart with this truth, Lord, so that I
remember this today. Be my refuge

from fear and discouragement about this weakness, and be my strength for this day. You *"are our refuge and strength, an ever-present help in times of trouble."* (Psalm 46:1, GOD'S WORD) I love you Lord, my strength. Amen.

weakness
prayer notes

_____

_____

_____

_____

_____

_____

_____

_____

_____

_____

_____

_____

_____

_____

healing

"Behold, I will bring to it health and healing, and I will heal them and reveal to them abundance of prosperity and security."
-Jeremiah 33:6-

Lord, as I cry out to you every day I beg you for healing from Lyme Disease, all of its co-infections, all of its complications, symptoms, and everything related to Lyme Disease. You are the great healer, Lord. God, it is you *"who forgives all of my sins and heals all my diseases"* (Psalm 103:3). Lord, Lyme disease has caused destruction and havoc on my body and on my life, but you can heal all of it. *"He sent his word and healed them, snatching them from the door of death."* (Psalm 107:20) You, and you alone can heal and restore my health just like I read you did when you walked here on earth. *"And Jesus went about all Galilee, teaching in their synagogues, and preaching the gospel of the kingdom, and healing all manner of sickness and all manner of disease among the people."* (Matthew 4:23) I cling to the promise Lord that you will restore my health to me and bring healing! *"For I will restore health to you, and I will heal you of your wounds…"* (Jeremiah 30:17) You are healing me even today Lord and I know that you are bringing health and healing to my body. *"Nevertheless, I will bring health and healing to it; I will heal my people and will let them enjoy abundant peace and security."* (Jeremiah 33:6) Amen.

healing
prayer notes

_____

_____

_____

_____

_____

_____

_____

_____

_____

_____

_____

_____

_____

_____

pain

"…Heal me, LORD, for my bones are
in agony."
-Psalm 6:2-

Lord, I am faint from the pain that is
deep within my body. It hurts, Lord, to
even take a breath. I would cry, but the
pain is so great that I have no tears left.
I am left with only a soul wrenching
agony of pain. *"Surely you are my help; you
are the one who sustains me."* (Psalm 54:4)
Because you sustain me, Lord, I will cry
out to you in my pain and beg you for
relief. With each breath that I take I cry
out for help saying, "Jesus, help me".
*"My body and mind may waste away (due to
the pain of this disease), but you, God, remain
the foundation of my life and my inheritance
forever."* (Psalm 73:26, GOD'S WORD)
In my pain today and in painful and
painless days ahead, *"it is good to be near
you God. I have made you, the Sovereign Lord,
my refuge."* (Psalm 73:28)I am crying out

in pain Lord. *"Be merciful to me, O Lord, for I am calling on you constantly."* (Psalm 86:2) Amen.

pain
prayer notes

_____

_____

_____

_____

_____

_____

_____

_____

_____

_____

_____

_____

_____

discouragement

"…This is what the LORD says to you:
Do not be afraid or discouraged because
of this vast army. For the battle is not
yours, but God's."
-2 Chronicles 20:15-

Lord, so often in this fight against
Lyme disease I find myself discouraged.
I know that you say in scripture to be
strong and courageous *"This is my
command- be strong and courageous! Do not be
afraid or discouraged. For the Lord your God
is with you wherever you go."* (Joshua 1:9)
You say not to be discouraged, but I
constantly am. Between the physical
symptoms and the emotional toll that
Lyme disease takes on my body, I find
myself more discouraged then hopeful.
Lord, you promise that *"you will fight for
me and that I only need to be still".* (Exodus
14:14) In another version of Exodus
14:14 you say, *"The LORD himself will
fight for you. Just stay calm."* You also

35

promise that this battle that I face is not mine alone, but yours. (2 Chronicles 20:15) Be with me, Lord, as I feel so discouraged each day. Give me the strength to rely on your promise that you are with me in each minute and each day. I can wake up with confidence each day that you are with me, and that you have this completely in control. *"But you will not even need to fight. Take your positions; then stand still and watch the LORD's victory. He is with you... do not be afraid or discouraged."*(2 Chronicles 20:17) You promise that my faith in you, Lord, will uphold me. (2 Chronicles 20:20) Give me peace for my discouragement, Lord, as I rest in the promise of your word. Amen.

discouragement
prayer notes

_____

_____

_____

_____

_____

_____

_____

_____

_____

_____

_____

_____

_____

_____

anger

" In your anger do not sin. Do not let
the sun go down while you are still
angry..."
-Ephesians 4:26-

Lord, sometimes in this journey I feel
nothing but absolute anger at what has
happened to my body. I am angry at this
disease, I am angry at how my life has
been affected by this disease, and I am
angry that I must walk this path set
before me. And sometimes, Lord, if I
am brutally honest I am even angry with
you that you have allowed this to
happen. Lord, I don't want to be angry.
I don't want to waste the precious
energy that I have being angry at
anything, especially not at you. You
have allowed this, but you are good,
Lord, and I choose not to be angry at
You. For if I stay angry, Lord, I am only
a fool. Scripture says, *"a fool gives full vent
to his anger, but a wise man holds it in check"*

(Proverbs 29:11). It also says, *"Do not be quickly provoked in your spirit, for anger resides in the lap of fools"* (Ecclesiastes 7:9). I don't want to be a fool. Take my anger, Lord, and place it at the foot of where it belongs- the truth that this is my temporary home. While bad things happen you are still God and I release the lie that I should find anger at you. Help me, Lord, to release this and to use that energy to fall more in love with who you are. Thank you for being a merciful and loving God who listens to all of my emotions and reminds me to not let the devil have a foothold by holding on to anger. (Ephesians 4:26) What an amazing God that you are that you care about all of me- including my hurts and anger. Amen.

anger
prayer notes

_____

_____

_____

_____

_____

_____

_____

_____

_____

_____

_____

_____

_____

_____

_____

fear

"So you have not received a spirit that
makes you fearful slaves."
-Romans 8:15-

Lord, one of the things I struggle most
with on this journey is the feelings of
fear over my current condition, and also
of what the future will look like. I know
that you say in Scripture that I have not
received a spirit that makes me a slave
to fear (Romans 8:15) but I am often in
terror of what may come. What if my
symptoms grow worse? What if I never
beat this disease? What if I spend the
rest of my life in bed? What if the pain
never subsides? What if something
happens to my caregiver? What if…
what if… what if… These questions
constantly plague my mind. I cling to
the verse that says, *"But now, this is what
the LORD says— he who created you, O
Jacob, he who formed you, O Israel: "Fear not,
for I have redeemed you; I have summoned you*

by name; you are mine. When you pass through the waters, I will be with you; and when you pass through the rivers, they will not sweep over you. When you walk through the fire, you will not be burned; the flames will not set you ablaze. For I am the LORD, your God, the Holy One of Israel, your Savior; Do not be afraid, for I am with you; Forget the former things; do not dwell on the past. See, I am doing a new thing! Now it springs up; do you not perceive it? I am making a way in the desert and streams in the wasteland." (Isaiah 43:1-5, 18, 19) Please, Lord, relieve my fears and help me know the truth of these verses deep within my soul. Let me be as strong as Joshua when he commanded those under him, *"Do not be afraid, do not be discouraged. Be strong and courageous."* (Joshua 10:25) I leave my fears in your hands, Lord. You are with me. I have nothing to fear for today or for the future. Amen.

fear
prayer notes

_____

_____

_____

_____

_____

_____

_____

_____

_____

_____

_____

_____

_____

_____

envy

"They seem to live such painless lives;
their bodies are so healthy and strong."
-Psalm 73:4-

Lord, as I struggle to even sit up in bed or get out of bed each day I envy those around me who do not have to deal with any health issues. From my vantage point Lord it seems that *"they have no struggles and their bodies are healthy and strong."* (Psalm 73:4) As I watch people go blithely on their way or listen to the complaints of those with no health issues I envy the cavalier approach to their health. I envy that they do not have to be constantly watching their health. I envy that *"they are free from common human burdens"* (Psalm 73:5). I envy *"that they are not plagued by human ills."* (Psalm 73:5) But Lord when I live in envy I miss the blessings that you have given me. I am not just this disease, and your blessings abound in this life you have given me. *"You, Lord, indeed will give what is good."* (Psalm 85:12)You, *"LORD, pour down your blessings."* (Psalm 85:12) Help me to focus on this and not be caught up in envy that will only lead to destruction. I know the truth of Proverbs 14: *"A tranquil heart makes for a healthy body, but jealousy is like bone cancer."* (Proverbs 14:30, GOD'S WORD) Amen.

envy
prayer notes

_____

_____

_____

_____

_____

_____

_____

_____

_____

_____

_____

_____

_____

financial stress

"So don't worry about these things, saying, 'what will we eat? What will we drink? What will we wear? These things dominate the thoughts of unbelievers, but your heavenly Father already knows all your needs. Seek the Kingdom of God above all else, and live righteously, and he will give you everything you need."
-Matthew 6:31-33-

Lord, as I find great comfort in knowing that the topic of money is addressed over 2,000 times in the Bible and that while on earth you spoke about this topic more than any other. You understand the heart of us humans so well, Lord. You understand that we worry about finances and I do worry about finances, Lord. It is hard to explain, Lord, the deep fear that I will not be able to provide for my basic needs let alone the treatment that I need to have to get better. Lord, I know that *"no one can serve two masters… I cannot serve both God and money."* (Matthew 6:24) And when I do not fully trust You to provide, Lord, then I am not serving you. You promise, Lord, that *"you will never fail me and never abandon me"* (Hebrews 13:5), and I trust that, Lord. Lord, help me to live in the truth of Matthew 6: *"If God gives such attention to the appearance of wildflowers- most of which are never even seen- don't you think He'll attend to you, do the best for you?"* (Matthew 6:31, THE MESSAGE) Amen.

financial stress prayer notes

_____

_____

_____

_____

_____

_____

_____

_____

_____

_____

_____

_____

_____

strength for treatment

"The Lord thy God in the midst of thee is mighty, He will save, He will rejoice over thee with joy…rest in His love, He will joy over thee with singing."
-Zephaniah 3:17-

Lord, if I thought being "sick" before the official diagnosis with Lyme was bad, I had no idea how difficult the treatment would be. I find myself so sick that I can't talk, my pain is excruciating, and I am afraid that I won't make it through. I need you Lord more than I ever have before. My prayer is that with each medication, supplement, or treatment there would be no adverse reactions, Lord, only help. You, Lord, are here and I do believe that You are mighty and that you will save. (Zephaniah 3:17) Lord, you promise that *"God is within her, she will not fall. God will help her at break of day."* (Psalm 46:5) Lord, help me believe this and know that you will give strength to endure and make it through treatment. My hope rests solely in you, Lord. *"Yet this I call to mind and therefore I have hope; Because of the Lord's great love we are not consumed, for His compassions never fail. They are new every morning; great is your faithfulness."* (Lamentations 3:21-24) You have never failed me, Lord. You are ever faithful. I will rest in your love and strength today. Amen.

strength for treatment prayer notes

_____

_____

_____

_____

_____

_____

_____

_____

_____

_____

_____

_____

_____

_____

loneliness

"Turn to me and be gracious to me, for
I am lonely and afflicted."
-Psalm 25:16-

Lord, sometimes it is not a big event
that brings out the intense feelings of
loneliness, as much as it is the day to
day things that remind me how alone I
truly am. Whether it is because I am
stuck in bed all day or whether it is
hearing about the latest coffee date I
had to miss out on, my heart is heavy
with loneliness. *"Turn to me, and have pity
on me. I am lonely and oppressed."* (Psalm
25:16, GOD'S WORD) You promise,
Lord, that *"you set the lonely in families, and
lead for the prisoners with singing..."* (Psalm
68:6) I am lonely, Lord, and I long to be
set in a family and lead the singing.
Lord, please heal my loneliness. Let my
heart be found solely in You because
You know me, Lord. You know all of
me. *"O LORD, you have examined my heart*

and know everything about me." (Psalm 139:1) And Lord, you don't just know me. You have chosen me. *"For you are a people holy to the Lord your God. Out of all of the peoples on the face of the earth, the Lord has chosen you to be His treasured possession."* (Deuteronomy 14:2) And because you know me and have chosen me I am never truly alone Lord. I rest in the truth of these promises. No matter my feelings, I am never alone because You are with me. Amen.

loneliness
prayer notes

_____

_____

_____

_____

_____

_____

_____

_____

_____

_____

_____

_____

_____

_____

feeling forsaken

"My God, my God, why have you
forsaken me? Why are you so far from
saving me, from the words of my
groaning?"
-Psalm 22:1-

Lord, with everything that has happened
in this illness journey, I struggle to not
feel forsaken by You. On the most
difficult days I cry out with the psalmist,
*"My God, my God, why have you abandoned
me? Why are you so far away when I groan for
help?"* (Psalm 22:1) In grief I cry out,
*"The Lord has forsaken me, my Lord has
forgotten me."* (Isaiah 49:14) As my grief
threatens to overwhelm me you quietly
and lovingly answer me Lord. You say
to my hurting heart: *"…For I have chosen
you and will not throw you away"* .(Isaiah
41:9) You remind me, Lord, that I am
worth more than the sparrows that you
take care of. *"Are not five sparrows sold for
two pennies? Yet not one of them is forgotten by*

God. Indeed, the very hairs of your head are all numbered. Don't be afraid; you are worth more than many sparrows." (Luke 12:6-7) You have not forsaken me, Lord. You are always with me. You promise, *"I will never leave you nor forsake you"* (Deuteronomy 31:6) and it is that truth I cling to, no matter how I feel. Amen.

feeling forsaken
prayer notes

_____

_____

_____

_____

_____

_____

_____

_____

_____

_____

_____

_____

_____

_____

_____

loss of who i was

"How can we sing the songs of the Lord
while in a foreign land?"
-Psalm 137:4-

Lord, the God who knows me even
when I don't recognize myself or my
life, I come to you knowing that You,
Lord, are unchanging. You, precious
Savior *"are the same yesterday, today, and
forever".* (Hebrews 13:8) Remind me,
Lord, when I feel dizzy with the changes
that this disease has brought that *you*
have not changed. Bring to mind the
truth of Scripture and who You are,
Lord. Help me to cling to the truth that
there is no circumstance that is touching
my life that you have not allowed or
deemed best for me. When the waves of
despair for all that this disease has taken
sweep over me, guide me, Lord, into
your truth. My heart cries out with the
psalmist who wrote, *"How can we sing a
song to the LORD on foreign soil?"* (Psalm

137:4). I feel that every single day. I am walking in a foreign land, Lord. My life might look vastly different then it was or what I planned for it to be, but I rest in peace knowing that You, Lord, never change, no matter what soil I am standing on- familiar or foreign- you are the place that I go to. *"Thou hast been our dwelling place throughout all generations."* (Psalm 90:1) The land where I live may change, but you never do. *"You are my refuge; my portion in the land of the living".* (Psalm 141:5) Amen.

loss of who i was
prayer notes

comparing the past to the present

"Do not say 'why were the old days betters than these' for it is not wise to ask such questions."
-Ecclesiastes 7:10-

Lord, if there is one battle that I fight with my mind all of the time, it is the temptation to allow the past to be better than today. It is so easy to compare life as of now to the one that I had before Lyme. Lord, You say in Scripture: *"Don't long for the good old days. This is not wise."* (Ecclesiastes 7:10) To be honest Lord I am not sure why except for the fact that by living in those questions I miss the blessings of the present. Lord, You promise, and *"I believe I shall look upon the goodness of the LORD in the land of the living."* (Psalm 27:13) Living is not in the past but in the present. Lord, You are the God of the past and I thank you for all of the wonderful memories and experiences that I had in the past. Even for the things that I didn't thank You for at the time, but now recognize as joy. Thank you. Lord, I am content though with where You have me now. There was life before Lyme but there is life after the diagnosis of Lyme disease. Show me, Lord, the way to live so that I remain humbly grateful for the past, but can view the present as the gift that it is.

Amen.

comparing the past to the present prayer notes

_____

_____

_____

_____

_____

_____

_____

_____

_____

_____

_____

_____

_____

_____

grief over the way i envisioned life to be like

"I will repay you for the years the
locusts have stolen..."
-Joel 2:28-

Lord, this is not how I envisioned my
life, at my age to look like. In my wildest
dreams this would have been farther
than I could have ever imagined. I long
for _____ and instead I am
on my sickbed. I am in grief, Lord, grief
over the way I envisioned life to be like.
I am grieving. Scripture promises that
*"Needy people will not always be forgotten.
Nor will the hope of oppressed people be lost
forever."* (Psalm 9:18, GOD'S WORD) I
am definitely needy, Lord, and I know
that you have not forgotten me. Lord,
while my days are not what I envisioned
or dreamed right now, I know that you
will repay the years that this disease has
stolen from me. You promise, *"I'll make
up for the years of the locust, the great locust*

devastation- locusts savage, locusts deadly, fierce locusts, locusts of doom, that great locust invasion I sent your way. You'll eat your fill of good food. You'll be full of praises to your God, the God who sent you back on your heels in wonder. Never again will my people be despised. You'll know without question that I'm in the thick of life with Israel, that I'm your God. Yes, You're God, the one and only real God." (Joel 2:25-27) And I rest in this promise, Lord, and in the peace of knowing that while I might never have dreamt this for my life but, *"I trust in you LORD, I say, 'You are my God'. My times are in your hands…"* (Psalm 31:14-15) Amen.

grief over the way i envisioned life to be like prayer notes

_____

_____

_____

_____

_____

_____

_____

_____

_____

_____

_____

_____

_____

_____

grief over loss of friends

"Scorn has broken my heart and has
left me helpless; I looked for sympathy,
but there was none, for comforters, but
I found none."
-Psalm 69:20-

Lord, you know the heartbreak that I
am experiencing right now as I have lost
friends. My heart is broken as I feel like
I have experienced death ten times over
as friends have walked away. Lord, You
know that *"reproach has broken my heart
and I am so sick. And I looked for sympathy,
but there was none. And for comforters, but I
found none."* (Psalm 69:20) Lord, mend
my heart and heal it. *"The LORD is near
to the brokenhearted and saves those crushed in
spirit."* (Psalm 34:18) so I know that you
will comfort me and save me. *"You heal
the brokenhearted and bind up their wounds"*
(Psalm 147:3). I cling to this promise,
Lord, that You will heal this gaping
wound in my heart. *"Because you are my*

help, I will sing in the shadow of your wings."
(Psalm 63:7) Amen.

grief over loss of friends prayer notes

_____

_____

_____

_____

_____

_____

_____

_____

_____

_____

_____

_____

grief over loss of family

"…Can a mother forget the baby at her breast and have no compassion on the child she has borne? Though she may forget, I will not forget you! See, I have engraved you on the palms of my hands…"
-Isaiah 49:15-16-

Lord, my grief is heavy as I am experiencing a wound so deep words can't even speak the depth of my loss. I am at a loss for words. I only have tears. I have been left alone, as the family member (or members) that I expected to walk with this journey with me, is unable or unwilling to do so. *"I have become estranged from my brothers and an alien to my mother's sons."* (Psalm 68:9) I feel like an alien, Lord. I have been abandoned. Lord, You promise that *"you are close to the brokenhearted"* (Psalm 34:18) and I am completely brokenhearted. This wound has pierced and shattered my heart. I don't know how to move forward from this point. All I can do is beg you for healing, Lord. Help me to remember that it is You, Lord, no one else that will walk this journey with me. *"It is God who arms me with strength and makes my way perfect."* (Psalm 18:32) No matter who leaves me on this journey, Lord, I am never alone because you are with me. *"Though my father and mother forsake me, the Lord will receive me."* (Psalm 27:10) You will never abandon me because you have engraved me on the palms of your hands! *"Can a mother forget the baby at her breast and have no compassion on the child she has borne? Though she may forget, I will not forget you! See, I have engraved you on the palms of my hands…"* (Isaiah 49:15-16) Another version states, *"Even if my father and mother abandon me, the LORD, will hold me close."* (Isaiah 49:15) Our grief in loss of those who leave overwhelms us, but you will never abandon us. Amen.

grief over loss of family
prayer notes

_____

_____

_____

_____

_____

_____

_____

_____

_____

_____

_____

_____

_____

grief over lack of understanding

"There is one whose rash words are like
sword thrusts…."
-Proverbs 12:18-

Lord, you know the heartbreak when
hasty words are spoken to me and show
a lack of understanding of what I am
dealing with in regards to this disease.
"Some people make cutting remarks…"
(Proverbs 12:18) Sometimes I think that
people are trying to give encouragement
but are not sure what to say. Other
times the words seem purposefully
hurtful. Either way, the lack of
understanding cuts to my heart. Truly,
Lord, *"Death and life are in the power of the
tongue…"* (Proverbs 18:21) Words that
are all too common that I and others
hear speak "death" and not "life" to my
situation. Help me to forgive those who
have hurt me with their words, Lord.
Help me to remember that my own
words have the power of life and death.

Lord, teach me to not speak death over my situation or another's situation. *"Let everything I say be good and helpful so that my words will be an encouragement to those who hear them."* (Ephesians 4:29). You are the God of life and I pray that my heart would overflow and speak this truth. *"May the words of my mouth and the meditation of my heart be pleasing to you, O LORD, my rock and my redeemer."* (Psalm 19:14) Amen.

grief over lack of understanding prayer notes

forgiveness

"And when you stand praying, if you hold anything against anyone, forgive them, so that your Father in heaven may forgive you your sins."
-Mark 11:25-

Lord, You state in Scripture that we are to forgive others. You state in Ephesians that we should *"get rid of all bitterness, rage, anger, harsh words, and slander…Instead, be kind to each other, tenderhearted, forgiving one another, just as God, has forgiven you."* (Ephesians 4:31-32) I know, Lord, that there are studies done that show links between health issues and un-forgiveness and I believe in your word, You speak about forgiving others. We are to *"forgive as you have forgiven us".* (Colossians 3:13) I don't want to hold onto anything that might detriment my healing, Lord, including un-forgiveness. Please help me to forgive those who have hurt me (whether in the past or in the present) and help me to place them in your care, Lord. Please forgive my own sins that I commit. Thank You for your grace and forgiveness in my life, Lord. It is amazing how You have forgiven me. Your love shouts of great love that I can share with others through forgiveness. Thank you, Lord. Amen.

forgiveness
prayer notes

_____

_____

_____

_____

_____

_____

_____

_____

_____

_____

_____

_____

_____

_____

the battle that never ends

"… the Lord has heard my weeping.
The Lord has heard my cry for
mercy…"
-Psalm 6:8-9-

*"Have compassion on me, LORD, for I am
weak. Heal me, LORD, for my bones are in
agony."* (Psalm 6:2) This battle, Lord,
seems never-ending. Each night as I lay
awake I weep with longing to be healed.
*"I am worn out from sobbing. All night I flood
my bed with weeping, drenching it with my
tears. My vision is blurred by grief..."* (Psalm
6:6-7) Like the Psalmist, Lord, I look at
this battle with this awful disease and
*"my soul is in deep anguish. How long
LORD, how long?"* (Psalm 6:3) will this
illness last? Please, Lord, turn to me.
Hear my cry and my supplication. *"Turn
LORD and deliver me; save me because of your
unfailing love."* (Psalm 6:4) Thank you,
Lord that my prayers are not in vain.
Thank You, *"Lord that you have heard the*

sound of my crying." (Psalm 6:8) Thank You, Lord, that you *have heard my plea; You accept my prayer."* (Psalm 6:8-9) Amen.

the battle that never ends
prayer notes

_____

_____

_____

_____

_____

_____

_____

_____

_____

_____

_____

_____

_____

_____

hope

"O Israel, hope in the LORD; for with
the LORD there is unfailing love. His
redemption overflows."
-Psalm 130:7-

Lord, hope is a waning thing as the
days grow longer with suffering. I find
myself questioning what I hope for and
what my hope is placed on. If it is on
healing, Lord, that is not enough. My
hope must be placed completely and
solely on You. *"We put our hope in the
LORD. He is our help and our shield. In
Him our hearts rejoice, for we trust in His
Holy name. Let your unfailing love surround
us, Lord, for our hope is in You."* (Psalm
33:30-22) As I put my hope in you
alone, Lord, I know that I will find
unfailing love. (Psalm 130:7) My hope is
secure in you, Lord. *"For I know the plans
I have for You, declares the Lord, Plans to
prosper you and not to harm you, plans to give
you hope and a future."* (Jeremiah 29:11)

"That is why we never give up. Though our bodies are dying, our spirits are being renewed every day. For our present troubles are small and won't last long. Yet they produce for us a glory that vastly outweighs them and will last forever! So we don't look at the troubles we can see now; rather, we fix our gaze on things that cannot be seen. For the things we see now will soon be gone, but the things we cannot see will last forever." (2 Corinthians 4:16-18) Amen.

hope
prayer notes

_____

_____

_____

_____

_____

_____

_____

_____

_____

_____

_____

_____

_____

_____

_____

_____

purpose in our pain

"Blessed be the God and Father of our Lord Jesus Christ, the Father of mercies and God of all comfort, who comforts us in all of our affliction, so that we may be able to comfort with which we ourselves are comforted by God."
-2 Corinthians 1:3-4-

Lord, in the midst of this battle with Lyme disease I find myself at a loss of what my purpose could possibly be. I feel so weak myself that the thought of finding a "great big purpose" in this pain is not only overwhelming, but seemingly impossible. There are so many days where I can't do anything but lay in bed. What purpose could be found there? But Lord, I also look around and I see there are so many hurting people just like myself. I see the vast multitudes of the brokenhearted- not only physically, but emotionally as well. You, Lord, are *"the Father who is compassionate and the God who gives comfort. You comfort us whenever we suffer. That is why whenever other people suffer,, we are able to comfort them by using the same comfort we have received from God.* (2 Corinthians 1:3-4, GOD'S WORD). Lord, You are the great comforter. Show me each day the purpose in my pain and this illness. Show me who I can comfort as you have comforted me. Show me who needs your love Lord, and how I can share it with them. And on days where I can only lay in bed, remind me to use that time to pray. There is always purpose to be found. Show me today what purpose there is in this story. Thank you Lord. Amen.

purpose in our pain
prayer notes

_____

_____

_____

_____

_____

_____

_____

_____

_____

_____

_____

_____

_____

desires of my heart

"May He give you the desires of your heart and make all of your plans succeed. May we shout for joy… May the Lord grant all of your requests."
-Psalm 20:4-5-

Lord, it seems that on this journey I have had to give up so many hopes, dreams, and desires for the future. Specifically, my immediate future. I see my dream of _____ passing me by, and it breaks my heart. You promise, Lord, that if we *"take delight in You, You will give us the desires of our hearts".* (Psalm 37:4) I want to delight in You alone, Lord, but sometimes my desires and dreams for my future seem to loom before me and take my eyes off of you. Give me your heart, Lord. Comfort me. I pray that you would take my eyes off of the thing (or things) that I think I am missing and put my attention back on you completely. When

I see others getting things that I desperately long for, help to me rejoice with them knowing that you are working in both of our lives according to your perfect will. (Romans 12:15) This is not about losing the desires of my heart, Lord, it is about surrendering to your love and your plans. I do, that, Lord with open hands. *"For the Lord is good. His unfailing love continues forever, and His faithfulness continues to each generation."* (Psalm 119:68) And *"the Lord is good and your love endures forever."* (Psalm 100:5) You are good, and I trust You completely with my deepest desires and longings. Amen.

desires of my heart
prayer notes

_____

_____

_____

_____

_____

_____

_____

_____

_____

_____

_____

_____

_____

_____

taking one day at a time

"So don't be anxious about tomorrow.
God will take care of your tomorrow
too. Live one day at a time."
-Matthew 6:34, THE MESSAGE-

Lord, help me to remember that on
this journey of life all I need to do is
take one day at a time. You say in
Scripture, *"don't be anxious about tomorrow.
God will take care of your tomorrow too. Live
one day at a time"* (Matthew 6:34) and I
want to do that, Lord. Sometimes all I
can see is the pain, the difficulty of this
disease, and all of the symptoms that I
am experiencing. It is hard to remember
that all we have is today. I put my
hopes, my concerns, and my fears in
your hands, Lord. *"Cast your cares on the
Lord and He will sustain you; He will never
let the righteous be shaken."* (Psalm 55:22) I
am casting my cares on you Lord. I
know that you can handle all of my fears
for what tomorrow may bring. You

promise to cover us, Lord, and to be our shield. *"He will cover you with His feathers, and under His wings you will find refuge; His faithfulness will be your shield and rampart."* (Psalm 91:4) All I have is today, Lord. The future is in your hands. I have no fear because You promise, Lord, that You are not only here today but with me tomorrow. *"The Lord is there."*(Ezekiel 48:35) Amen.

taking one day at a time
prayer notes

_____

_____

_____

_____

_____

_____

_____

_____

_____

_____

_____

_____

_____

choosing joy

"Today I have given you the choice
between life and death, between
blessings and curses. Now I call on
heaven and earth to witness the choice
you make. Oh, that you would choose
life, so that you, and your descendants
might live."
-Deuteronomy 30:19-

Lord, today, despite all of the symptoms
of Lyme disease, all of the side effects of
treatment, and all of the health issues, I
want to choose life. I want to choose
joy. You say, *"today I place before you life
and death, blessing and curse. Choose life so
that you and your children will live. And love
God, your God, listening obediently to Him,
firmly embracing Him. Oh yes, He is life itself,
a long life settled…"* (Deuteronomy 30:19,
THE MESSAGE) Lord, I want to
choose life in this situation even though
I feel so terrible. I know that in
choosing life I will be choosing joy. You

say in Scripture to *"consider it pure joy…
whenever you face trials of many kinds, because
you know that the testing of your faith develops
perseverance"* (James 1:2-3) and, Lord, that
perseverance is reminding me that all
joy, no matter the circumstances is
found only in you. Lord, *"the hope of the
righteous is joy"* (Proverbs 10:28) and that
is where I find my joy completely. Help
me, Lord, even on the darkest of days in
this journey, to choose joy. Amen.

choosing joy
prayer notes

_____

_____

_____

_____

_____

_____

_____

_____

_____

_____

_____

_____

_____

_____

_____

hope for the future

"She is clothed with strength and dignity, and she laughs without fear of the future."
-Proverbs 31:25-

Lord, sometimes I look at my reflection in the mirror and I don't know the person staring back at me. So much has changed physically, emotionally, and mentally in this journey. I sometimes long for life to be "normal", and yet I have no idea what "normal" would look like anymore. Let my fears, my hopes, my longings, and my hope for the future be solely found in you. Let my wisdom for the future come from you alone. *"In the same way, wisdom is sweet to your soul. If you find it, you will have a bright future, and your hopes will not be cut short."* (Proverbs 24:14) My faith for my future hope rests solely on You, Lord. You will lead me each step of the way- through this journey – and beyond it. I am confident, Lord, that you have a plan, a plan *"for welfare and not for evil, to give me a future and a hope"* (Jeremiah 29:11). And that is what I rest in today, Lord. The plan and the promise that I can't see yet, but in You, the one who loves me more than life. *"Faith is the confidence that what we hope for will actually happen; it gives us assurance about things we cannot see."* (Hebrews 11:1) Amen.

hope for the future prayer notes

_____

_____

_____

_____

_____

_____

_____

_____

_____

_____

_____

_____

_____

_____

a note from rebecca

Sweet Friend,

When I first wrote "Praying through Lyme Disease" in 2014 I was really at the beginning stages of this journey. Oh, I thought I had experienced the worst days of this journey, but I was to find that there were still more difficult and more painful days to come than I could have ever imagined. But, as I conclude this second edition, I look back with gratitude and see that despite the horrors of this disease, the Lord, in His infinite mercy has always been incredibly kind. He has never once abandoned me, and in hundreds of big and small ways I see the answers to the prayers that are listed in this book.

I hope and pray that as you walk through this journey this book will be just a starting point of what to pray. I'm praying for you, dear friend, and I trust you'll be praying for me as well as we continue to fight the good fight and walk this journey before us. This journey is difficult, hard, messy, and extremely painful, and yet, can be full of hope as we experience the tender mercy of a faithful God who is walking every step with us.

May you experience and know His love in new ways throughout this Lyme disease journey.

You are not alone.
You are not forgotten.
You are truly seen.

With Love, Rebecca

index list of scripture references & versions

ACKNOWLEDGEMENTS
Psalm 66:16-20- New International Version

A NOTE FROM THE AUTHOR
Psalm 25:5- New International Version
Psalm 20:1-5- New International Version

THE DIAGNOSIS
Psalm 23:4- New Living Translation
Psalm 23:4- King James Version
Isaiah 52:12- New International Version
Isaiah 54:10- GOD'S WORD Translation

CONFUSION OVER TREATMENT OPTIONS

2 Timothy 2:7- English Standard Version

I Corinthians 14:33- English Standard Version

2 Corinthians 4:8- English Standard Version

Luke 10:19- King James Version

2 Timothy 2:7- English Standard Version

WISDOM FOR DOCTORS

James 1:5- GOD'S WORD Translation

James 1:5- English Standard Version

Proverbs 3:5-7- New International Version

Colossians 1:9- English Standard Version

Psalm 115:15- New International Version

FEELING DISCOURAGED OVER MEDICAL CARE
Mark 5:26- New Living Translation
Mark 5:26- English Standard Version
2 Chronicles 16:12- New International Version
John 5:1-9- New International Version

FEELING LIKE A BURDEN
Mark 2:4- New Living Translation
Psalm 55:22- New Living Translation

GUILT OVER HOW LITTLE I AM ABLE TO DO
I Peter 4:16- English Standard Version
Galatians 6:4- New Living Translation
Hebrews 12:1- New Living Translation
I Peter 4:16- New International Version

WEAKNESS
Deuteronomy 33:25- King James Version
Psalm 18:32- New International Version
Psalm 18:39- New International Version
Psalm 46:1- GOD'S WORD Translation

HEALING
Jeremiah 33:6- English Standard
Version
Psalm 103:3- New Living Translation
Psalm 107:20- New Living Translation
Matthew 4:23- King James Version
Jeremiah 30:17- New Living Translation
Jeremiah 33:6- New International
Version

PAIN
Psalm 6:2- New International Version
Psalm 54:4- New International Version
Psalm 73:26- GOD'S
WORD Translation
Psalm 73:28- New Living Translation
Psalm 86:3- New International Version

DISCOURAGEMENT
2 Chronicles 20:15- New International Version
Joshua 1:9- New Living Translation
Exodus 14:14- New International Version
Exodus 14:14- New Living Translation
2 Chronicles 20:20- New Living Translation

ANGER
Ephesians 4:26- New International Version
Proverbs 29:11- Holman Christian Standard Bible
Ecclesiastes 7:9- New International Version

FEAR
Romans 8:15- New Living Translation
Isaiah 43:1-5, 18-19- New International Version
Joshua 10:25- New International Version

ENVY
Psalm 73:4- New Living Translation
Psalm 73:4- New International Version
Psalm 73:5- New International Version
Psalm 85:12- New International Version
Psalm 85:12- New Living Translation
Proverbs 14:30- GOD'S
WORD Translation

FINANCIAL STRESS
Matthew 6:31-33- New Living
Translation
Matthew 6:24- New International
Version
Hebrews 13:5- New Living Translation
Matthew 6:31- The MESSAGE

STRENGTH FOR TREATMENT
Zephaniah 3:17- King James Version
Psalm 46:5- New International Version
Lamentations 3:21-24- New
International Version

LONELINESS
Psalm 25:16- New International Version
Psalm 25:16- GOD'S
WORD Translation
Psalm 68:6- New International Version
Psalm 139:1- New Living Translation
Deuteronomy 14:2- New International
Version

FEELING FORSAKEN
Psalm 22:1- English Standard Version
Psalm 22:1- New Living Translation
Isaiah 49:14- English Standard Version
Isaiah 41:9- New Living Translation
Luke 12:6-7- New International Version
Deuteronomy 31:6- New International
Version

LOSS OF WHO I WAS
Psalm 137:4- New International Version
Psalm 137:4- NET Bible
Psalm 90:1- King James Version
Psalm 141:5- King James Version

COMPARING THE PAST TO THE PRESENT
Ecclesiastes 7:10- New International Version
Ecclesiastes 7:10- New Living Translation
Psalm 27:13- English Standard Version

GRIEF OVER THE WAY I ENVISIONED LIFE TO BE LIKE
Joel 2:25- New International Version
Psalm 9:18- GOD'S WORD Translation
Joel 2:25-27- The MESSAGE
Psalm 31:14-15- New International Version

GRIEF OVER LOSS OF FRIENDS
Psalm 69:20- New International Version
Psalm 69:20- New American Standard Bible
Psalm 34:18- English Standard Version
Psalm 147:3- New International Version
Psalm 63:7- New International Version

GRIEF OVER LOSS OF FAMILY
Isaiah 49:15-16- New International
Version
Psalm 68:9- English Standard Version
Psalm 34:18- New International Version
Psalm 18:32- New Living Translation
Psalm 27:10- New International Version
Psalm 27:10- New Living Translation

GRIEF OVER LACK OF
UNDERSTANDING
Proverbs 12:18- English Standard
Version
Proverbs 12:18- New Living Translation
Proverbs 18:21- English Standard
Version
Ephesians 4:29- New Living Translation
Psalm 19:14- New International Version

FORGIVENESS
Mark 11:25- New International Version
Ephesians 4:31-32- New Living
Translation
Colossians 3:13- New Living
Translation

THE BATTLE THAT NEVER ENDS

Psalm 6:8-9- New International Version
Psalm 6:2- New Living Translation
Psalm 6:6-7- New Living Translation
Psalm 6:3- New Living Translation
Psalm 6:4- New International Version
Psalm 6:8- GOD'S WORD Translation
Psalm 6:9- English Standard Version

HOPE

Palm 130:7- New Living Translation
Psalm 33:20-22- New Living Translation
Jeremiah 29:11- New International Version
2 Corinthians 4:16-18- New Living Translation

PURPOSE IN OUR PAIN

2 Corinthians 1:3-4- English Standard Version
2 Corinthians 1:3-4- GOD'S WORD Translation

DESIRES OF MY HEART
Psalm 20:4-5- New International
Version
Psalm 37:4- New International Version
Psalm 119:68- New International
Version
Psalm 100:5- New Living Translation

TAKING ONE DAY AT A TIME
Matthew 6:34- The MESSAGE
Psalm 55:22- New International Version
Psalm 91:4- New International Version
Ezekiel 48:35- New International
Version

CHOOSING JOY
Deuteronomy 30:19- New Living
Translation
Deuteronomy 30:19- The MESSAGE
James 1:2-3- New International Version
Proverbs 10:28-New International
Version

HOPE FOR THE FUTURE
Proverbs 31:25- New Living Translation
Proverbs 24:14- New Living Translation
Hebrews 11:1- New Living Translation

about the author

Rebecca VanDeMark is a writer, speaker, and blogger who loves Jesus, life, and the miracle of hope. Rebecca is the author of five books, including, *"Praying through Lyme Disease"*. Rebecca holds degrees from Cedarville University, Regent University, and American University. Before fighting health issues Rebecca worked in Washington DC with two non-profit organizations and later taught High School History and Bible Classes for seven years. Rebecca loves celebrating the beauty of the ordinary each day as she fights Lyme disease in addition to other health issues. She lives with her family, splitting time between the sweet south and upstate New York.

Connect with Rebecca on a daily basis, see pictures, and follow her writing and speaking ministry:

Website: www.rebeccavandemark.com
Blog: www.caravansonnet.com
Instagram:
www.instagram.com/rebeccaannvande
mark
Facebook:
www.facebook.com/rebeccaannvandem
ark
Twitter:
www.twitter.com/caravansonnet
Email:
rebeccaannvandemark@gmail.com

---

i

http://www.mvlymecenter.org/2012/08/08/in-the-fullness-of-time/

ii

http://www.mvlymecenter.org/2012/08/08/in-the-fullness-of-time/

---

also available from Rebecca
coming November 2017
WHEN LYME INVADES
RELEASING NOVEMBER 1ST, 2017

WHEN LYME
INVADES

ENCOURAGEMENT AND PRACTICAL TIPS FOR
LOVING YOUR FRIEND THROUGH LYME DISEASE

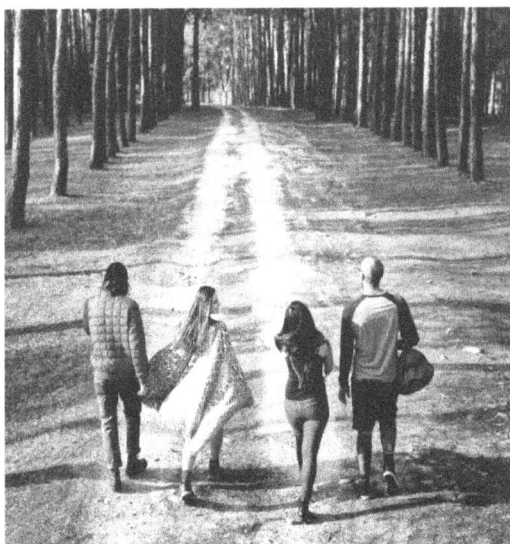

REBECCA VANDEMARK
AUTHOR OF PRAYING THROUGH LYME DISEASE

WHEN TRUTH REFRESHES
LARGE PRINT EDITION
RELEASING MAY 2018

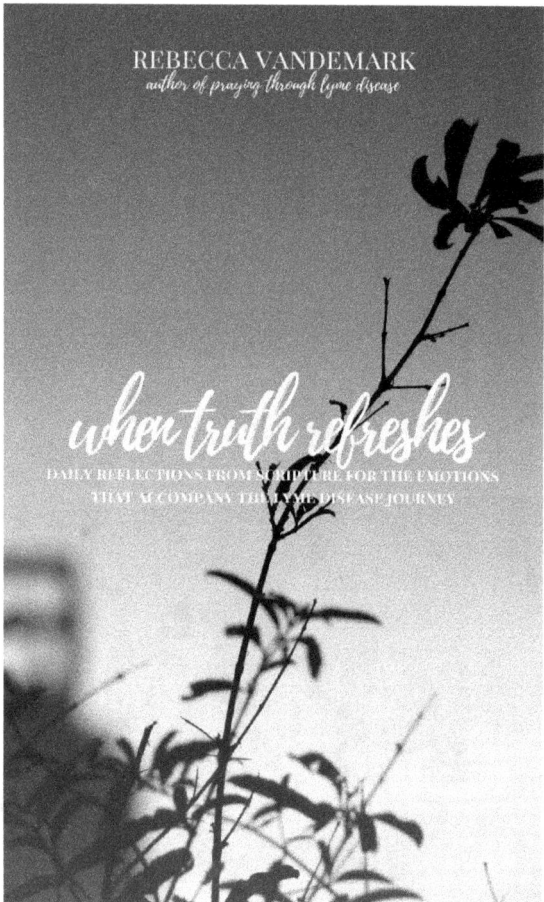

PATH OF HOPE
LARGE PRINT EDITION
RELEASING JULY 2017

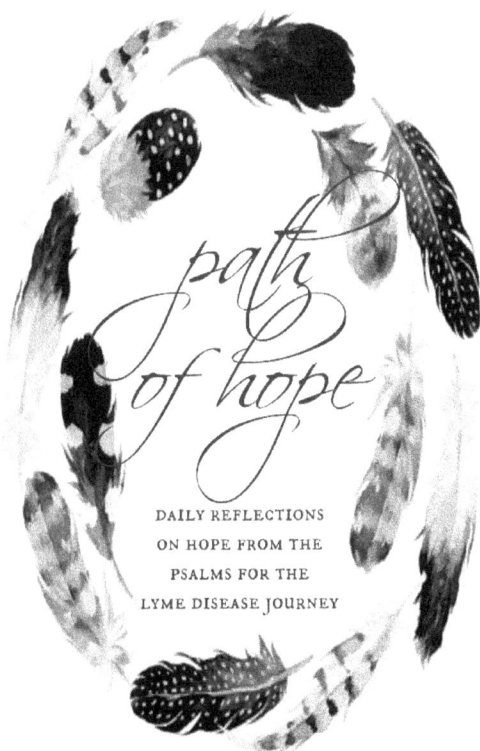

path
of hope

DAILY REFLECTIONS
ON HOPE FROM THE
PSALMS FOR THE
LYME DISEASE JOURNEY

REBECCA VANDEMARK
author of Praying Through Lyme Disease

WHEN LIGHT DAWNS
LARGE PRINT EDITION
RELEASING NOVEMBER 2018

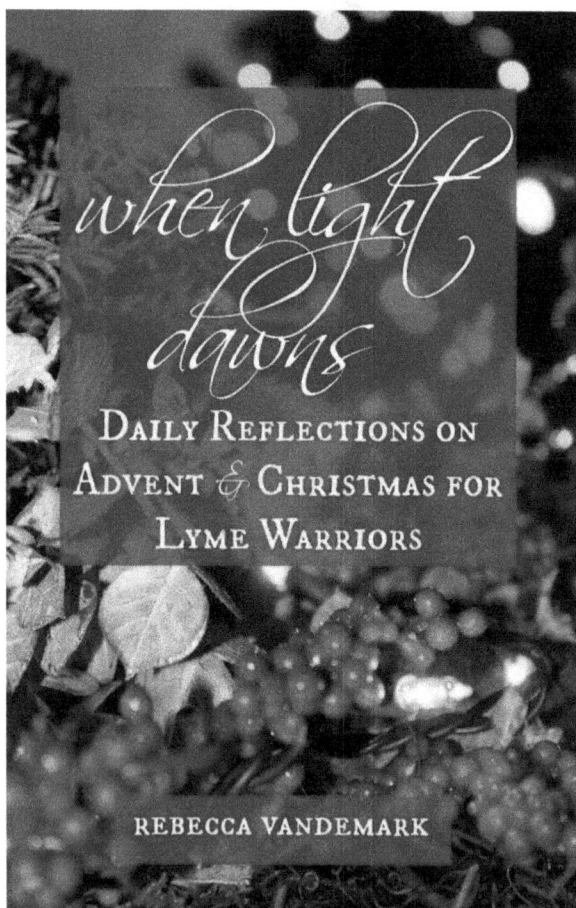